Guide on everything fat loss:
A practical solution to weight loss and muscle building

Albert D. Willer

Table of contents

Chapter 1

Losing weight is what?

Most of the time under the skin (subcutaneous) or in the bodily cavity (visceral), with a minor proportion, also being stored in our muscles, adipose tissue is where our bodies store fat (intramuscular). A source of stored energy is body fat.

The body recognizes when the molecules that give you energy are running low in your bloodstream and turns to its fat reserves for support.
Storage of fat and energy
In fat cells, fats are stored as triglycerides that are released by the hormone-sensitive lipase enzyme (HSL). Fatty acids can then enter the bloodstream and travel there while attached to a protein called albumin before entering muscles to be "burned." The term beta-oxidation also refers to the "burning" of fat.
Via this beta-oxidation, tissues may degrade fatty acids. ATP, the energy supply for cells, is eventually produced through the beta-oxidation process.
It occurs in the mitochondria. Carnitine allows fatty acids to enter the mitochondria.
There may not be an immediate requirement for fatty acids when large quantities are broken down and overwhelm the mitochondria (as in hunger). Ketones are the result in this instance, which are energy-dense

pieces. This is significant because, while fat cannot be turned into glucose, it may still give energy in the form of these ketones to the muscles and the brain.
flowchart for catabolism
The body uses the ATP produced from the breakdown of fat for metabolic functions including breathing, controlling body temperature, digesting, and excretion. We acquire around 70% of the ATP generated during rest and extremely low-intensity activity from lipids.

Why is weight loss so crucial?
We must shed this fat...
People in the majority of developed cultures are probably overweight as a whole.
2007-05-06-world-fatness
This issue goes beyond simple aesthetics. Nearly every aspect of life can be negatively impacted by excess body fat, including:
reduction in mobility
Organ failure risk is higher with lower emotional well-being and self-esteem.
worsening cardiovascular condition
heightened potential for heart illness
heightened potential for stress fractures
increased stroke risk
greater possibility of cancer
reduced sexual and reproductive fitness
The production of hormones by fat cells, which can function as endocrine factories, can affect a variety of bodily functions, most of which promote the storage of more body fat.

Beyond just being healthier, having less body fat is frequently viewed as being more beautiful and appealing since it reveals the underlying muscles.

For many athletes (apart from sumo wrestlers, linemen, etc.), having a lower body fat percentage is helpful since more fat weight generates drag and extra resistance that must be overcome.

The bottom fact is that having a lot of extra body fat negatively affects your health, body composition, and athletic performance.

But it's difficult.

But here's the issue: as a whole, we're also not very adept at shedding weight.

Less than 10% of patients who have bariatric surgery or use other current obesity treatments successfully maintain their weight permanently.

Approximately 95% of overweight people attempt many diets, only to put on the majority or all of the weight back within a year. Over 70% of Americans are overweight or obese. Since 1980, the proportion of overweight children aged 12 to 17 has risen.

A better answer is required. Understanding how fat loss occurs may be useful.

What you must understand

Body fat is mostly stored in fat cells, which are constantly changing. Nutritional, metabolic, and hormonal variables independently control how much fat is burned, which has an impact on both the amount of body fat and the amounts of circulating fatty acids.

hormones and weight loss

Lower insulin levels and an increase in the hormones glucagon, cortisol, adrenaline, and growth hormone are needed for fatty acid release and utilization. These hormones that are "anti-insulin" stimulate HSL. Thyroxine is a second important hormone that affects how fat is metabolized (thyroid hormone).

Glycogen is produced following a substantial meal until reserves are refilled. When blood sugar levels are too high, glucose is converted into fatty acids. Fatty acids can also be produced from amino acids. Lipoprotein lipase is the enzyme
required for triglyceride absorption by cells.
Insulin levels drop and anti-insulin hormone levels rise in the fasting state. This quickens the utilization of fat.

Loss of weight and calorie shortfall

When we drastically cut back on calories, the body is incredibly good at preserving our fat reserves.
Thyroid hormone synthesis is lowered because insulin levels are low. This lowers the metabolism during rest. Within 24 hours of beginning an intensive diet, this can happen.
After the diet is abandoned, rebound weight gain is all but guaranteed due to the body's reaction to calorie restriction. The body often gains more fat when the muscle is gone.
Fats serve as more than just a fuel source for low-intensity activity and periods of rest. Fats replenish phosphagens that have been depleted by vigorous

activity. The "afterburn" effect allows for a return to pre-exercise circumstances following prolonged, hard exercise sessions by increasing oxygen intake.
stages of fuel consumption when fasting
stages of fuel consumption when fasting
Fat loss is a challenging issue.

During the past 30 years, our emphasis on certain nutrients, intensive nutrition advice, dieting, and consumption of processed foods have all contributed to an increase in body fat. In other words, we have become fatter as a result of more information, diets, and junk food.
Even though part of this may appear counterintuitive, it serves as an example of the value of bodily awareness (hunger/satiety cues), avoiding processed meals, engaging in regular physical activity, and heeding food advertisements.

Chapter 2

What You Should Know Before You Start A Weight-loss Plan.

For personal reasons, you might desire to reduce your weight. Or perhaps you need to drop weight to get healthier. The chance of developing certain diseases, including heart disease and type 2 diabetes, can be decreased. Your blood pressure and overall cholesterol level may decrease as a result. Also, it might lessen the effects of the symptoms of being overweight and stop accidents.

Several things might interfere with your weight loss attempts. You may do this by altering your food, workout routine, and lifestyle. You can stay on track with the help of tools and advice. You should also be aware of what to avoid doing. Before you start a new strategy, consult your doctor.

They may assist you in modifying a program and securely tracking your advancement. Your health can be significantly improved by even little adjustments.

a way to better health
There are more tasks you should do before beginning. Stick to the diet and exercise regimen. Think about telling your loved ones. They can support you and assist

in keeping track of your development. This makes you answerable.

There are three crucial truths regarding weight loss. Your weight is the first. The second factor is your BMI (BMI). Your height and weight are used to calculate your BMI. BMI is regarded by doctors as the most accurate indicator of your health risk. In reality, the BMI scale is the basis for the medical words "overweight" and "obesity."

A BMI of 25 to 30 is regarded as overweight. A BMI of 30 or more is regarded as obese. The risk of a condition associated with excess weight increases with your BMI. Heart disease and type 2 diabetes are included in this. You may use a BMI calculator or consult your doctor to determine your BMI. Adults of both sexes can use the BMI chart. Under-20-year-old males and girls have their charts. Moreover, there is a BMI calculator specifically for Asian patients.

To lose weight, you need to be aware of your waist circumference. Your belly region is where body fat tends to accumulate. Compared to body fat that accumulates in your thighs or buttocks, this is a bigger health danger. Your waist circumference is a useful measurement because of this. Start by placing the tape measure's one end on top of your hip bone. Make sure the other end is straight when you wrap it around your midsection. Neither the tape nor its tension should be excessive.

Chapter 3.

What happens when a fat cell is burned?

The majority of individuals have little to no
 understanding of how fat cells function, how fat is
burned, or where burned fat goes. Even though it is a
very complicated physiological process, several
researchers and industry professionals attempted to
simplify it. When the body burns fat, the fat cell does not
leave the body or become a muscle cell. When body fat
is high, it is difficult to discern muscle "definition" since
the fat cell itself remains exactly where it was
underneath the skin in the thighs, hips, arms, etc., and
on top of the muscles (Porter et al., 2009).

Triacylglycerol, a type of fat, is kept inside fat cells. It
takes many intricate hormonal and enzymatic processes
for the fat to be released from the fat cell; it is not burnt
there in the fat cell.
Triacylglycerol is simply released by the fat cell into the
circulation as free fatty acids (FFAs) when it is prompted
to do so, and these FFAs are then carried by the blood
to the tissues where the energy is required (Manore et
al. 2011).

Each triglyceride molecule separates into glycerol and three fatty acids during lipolysis. The reaction that hormone-sensitive lipase catalyzes (HSL). When the muscles need energy, the FFAs that have been stored in the body are released into circulation.
More FFAs are supplied to the muscles that require them when blood flow to the active muscles rises. LPL allows FFAs to enter the mitochondria, where they are transported and burnt. The shrinking of the fat cell as a result of the release of FFAs from it is what gives the body its slimmer appearance when fat is lost (Fig. 3; Turcotte, 2000).

Scientists concluded that fat cells are similar to storage tanks and that we don't truly "lose" fat cells; rather, we "clear out" fat cells. Body fat is essentially simply a reserve source of energy.
The size of fat cells can change depending on how "full" they are, unlike a petrol tank in a car that is set in size (Robergs and Keteyian 2013). Humans continue to be leaner despite consuming more energy-dense foods and fats for a variety of reasons.

Why-do-slim-people-who-eat-lot-never-seem-put-wei ght):

1. Not just due to the traditional adage that they have a quicker metabolism than everyone else, but also due to their estimated total calorie consumption.
2. They slept 6 to 8 hours every night, consumed little to no soft drinks (avoiding excessive sugar contents),

rarely ate out (keeping processed foods to a minimum), ate meals sitting down (people who ate a meal standing up ate twice as much after they finished the food, considering the food to be a snack, not a meal), do not really snack a lot, and also incorporated an eating and exercise routine into their lives (meals were eaten at regular times during the day).

Chapter 4

Done fat loss means weight loss.

When you lose weight, your total body weight decreases as a result of muscle, water, and fat reductions.

In contrast to weight loss, which is more general and unhealthy, fat loss refers to weight reduction from fat.

It might be challenging to distinguish between muscle and fat loss, though.
This article discusses why losing fat is more significant than decreasing weight, how to distinguish between the two, and offers advice on how to lose fat while keeping muscle.

How to determine if you are losing weight
Using a scale to monitor your weight reduction progress is customary.

Although this is useful, most scales don't distinguish between muscle loss and fat loss.

Because of this, monitoring your weight alone is not a reliable way to ascertain whether you are losing muscle or fat, and if so, how much.

A body fat scale, on the other hand, can give you a more accurate picture of your body composition by calculating your ratio of fat to muscle.

Furthermore, skinfold calipers may be used to calculate your body fat %, although accuracy with this method requires practice

Chapter 5

What diet burns the fattest?

When someone starts a diet, they often decide whether to cut off carbohydrates or fat. Then they endure agonizing months of waiting, hoping that the route they took may enable them to lose a few dress sizes. The time for speculating may now be passed. A low-fat diet is a way to go if you want to lose the most weight, according to research supported by the National Institutes of Health. A low-carb diet, however, does reduce insulin levels and increases fat burning.

It's confusing, we admit. Here is an explanation: Kevin Hall, a researcher in metabolism at the National Institute of Diabetes and Digestive and Kidney Diseases, has been examining how the body reacts to two distinct diets since 2003: one where the fat intake was maintained while calories were reduced by 30% by eliminating carbohydrates, and the other where the exact opposite was true. Hall imprisoned 19 individuals for two weeks in a metabolic ward (with their cooperation) to conduct the study as accurately as feasible. Every meal was carefully monitored by the researchers.

Hall discovered that despite the mirror-image diet with fewer carbohydrates burning more fat, the diet with lower fat led to a larger total reduction of body fat. The amount of fat consumed and burned throughout each diet was assessed by the researchers, and the data were used to determine the study participants' rate of body-fat loss. Hall came to the additional conclusion that the body appears to lessen the disparities between a low-fat and a low-carb diet over time. Yet, his research recommends choosing a low-fat food plan while you are just beginning to diet.

According to one set of ideas, all calories are equally effective in reducing body fat, while another contends that cutting back on carbohydrates will increase fat loss.

Hall makes this point in an article published in the journal Cell Metabolism. Our findings demonstrated that, while not all calories are equally effective in reducing body fat, they come quite close over the long run.

Chapter 6

What to avoid when losing weight.

Certain foods are high in sugar, refined carbs, and fat, yet low in important nutrients like protein and fiber. This can make weight loss more difficult and may have other negative effects on health.

Most people who want to lose weight only reduce their calorie intake.

But you must also take into account the kinds of meals you're consuming.

Protein and fiber-rich foods can help you feel satisfied for longer, which may aid in weight reduction.
On the other side, consuming an excessive amount of meals heavy in fat, sugar, or refined carbohydrates might increase your calorie intake and make weight reduction more difficult.

These are 11 things you should avoid eating if you want to lose weight.

1. Potato chips with French fries

The calorie and fat content of potato chips and french fries is frequently extremely high.

Consuming potato chips and French fries has been associated with weight gain and obesity in observational studies.

A 2011 study indicated that, compared to other foods, potato chips may cause higher weight gain per serving. Moreover, acrylamides, which have been related to cancer, may be present in baked, roasted, or fried potatoes.

Summary
When taken in excess, potato chips, and french fries can cause weight gain since they are heavy in calories and fat. Hence it's advisable to just consume these things occasionally.

2. Sugary beverages

Sodas and other drinks with added sugar have a lot of calories.

When ingested in excess, they are strongly linked to weight gain and can be harmful to one's health. Sugary beverages include a lot of calories, yet your brain doesn't perceive them as real food. Since liquid sugar calories don't make you feel as satisfied, you won't cut back on your food intake to make up for them. Instead, you could find yourself consuming more calories than usual after adding them.

If you're serious about reducing weight, you might want to avoid drinking as much sugar-sweetened liquid and switch to flavored water, kombucha, tea, or coffee instead.

SUMMARY

Your weight and overall health might be significantly impacted by sugary beverages. Limiting your use of soda and other similar drinks may have a significant influence on your weight reduction efforts.

3. White bread

White bread is extremely processed and frequently loaded with added sugar.
It has a high glycemic index, which means that it may cause a fast rise in blood sugar levels
Eating two slices (120 grams) of white bread per day was associated with a 40% higher risk of weight gain and obesity, according to a 2014 study including 9,267 participants.

All wheat slices of bread do, however, contain gluten, which anyone with celiac disease or gluten sensitivity should avoid.

Other bread choices for people on a gluten-free diet include oopsie bread, cornbread, and bread made with almond flour.

SUMMARY
White bread's high glycemic index has been connected to obesity and weight gain. Moreover, it includes gluten, which may not be healthy for those who have celiac disease or gluten intolerance.

4. Sweets bars

Candy bars come in compact packaging with a lot of refined flour, added sugar, and additional oils.

Candy bars include few nutrients and a lot of calories. Several chocolate-covered candy bars kinds have between 200 and 300 calories per bar, and extra-large bars could have even more.

If you have a sweet tooth, go for a little candy bar or a few squares of dark chocolate and eat them with other healthy snacks like yogurt parfaits, fresh fruit, almonds, or candy bars.

SUMMARY
 Candy bars include a lot of sugar, processed flour, and extra oils. They have a lot of calories as well, but they don't fill you up.

5. A few juices of fruits.

Several of the fruit juices you may buy at the grocery store are significantly different from the actual fruit.

Some varieties can have at least as many calories and sugars as soda.
Fruit juice often has no fiber and doesn't need to be chewed.

This makes it possible to eat big amounts of orange juice in a short period because a glass won't have the same effects on fullness as an orange.

Use whole fruit instead, or try consuming no more than 4 ounces (118 milliliters) of fruit juice at a time.

SUMMARY
 Fruit juice often lacks fiber but is heavy in calories and added sugar. It is advisable to pick whole fruit or stick to smaller quantities.

5. Cakes, biscuits, and pastries

Cakes, cookies, and pastries are all high in calories and sugar.

Also, these high-calorie items are not very filling, which means that you can feel hungry again very soon after eating them.

If you're attempting to lose weight, consider consuming these meals in moderation and including them sometimes in a well-balanced diet.

Instead, you may try eating things like dark chocolate, berries, trail mix, or chia pudding.

SUMMARY
 Although heavy in calories and added sugar, pastries, cookies, and cakes are not especially satisfying. Choosing different sweet snacks or reducing your portion sizes may aid with weight management.

7. A few forms of alcohol (especially beer)

Around 7 calories per gram of alcohol are more calories than either protein or carbohydrates.
Yet, there are conflicting data linking alcohol use to weight gain.
Alcohol also has an impact. Beer can lead to weight gain, whereas moderate wine consumption may have health benefits.

SUMMARY
 If you're attempting to reduce weight, you might want to think about reducing your alcohol consumption or only drinking wine occasionally.

8. Ice cream

The majority of ice cream varieties are not only heavy in calories but also sugary.

Every once in a while, a modest serving of ice cream is great, but the issue is that it's incredibly simple to eat a lot of it all at once.

To avoid overeating, be careful to pour yourself a modest serving of ice cream rather than eating it directly from the carton.
As an alternative, think about preparing your frozen desserts with less sugar and healthier components like fruit and full-fat yogurt.

SUMMARY
Store-bought ice cream has a lot of calories and sugar. If you're attempting to lose weight, making your frozen treats at home with less sugar or sticking to fewer ice cream servings might be helpful.

9. Pizza

A particularly well-liked quick food is pizza. However, the components used to make professionally prepared pizzas, such as highly refined flour and processed meat, are frequently rich in calories.

Make your own at home using wholesome toppings and ingredients if you want to enjoy a piece of pizza.

Stick to lower-calorie toppings when ordering at a restaurant, such as grilled chicken, peppers, onions, spinach, mushrooms, or garlic.

To cut calories, you may also pick thin-crust pizza. To complete your meal, have a piece or two with a side of steamed broccoli or a salad.

SUMMARY
 Highly processed and refined materials are frequently used to make commercial pizzas. Cooking your pizza at home or choosing toppings with fewer calories might help you control your weight.

10. Caffeine-rich coffee beverages

Caffeine is one of several physiologically active ingredients in coffee.
At least temporarily, these substances can enhance your metabolism and fat burning.

Yet, excessive quantities of cream and sugar in many coffee beverages can considerably raise the number of calories in each cup.

Choosing basic, black coffee that has been lightly sweetened with some cream or milk is preferable if you're attempting to lose weight.

SUMMARY
Your metabolism may be boosted and fat burning increased by drinking plain, black coffee. Unfortunately, a lot of coffee beverages have too much sugar and cream, which might raise the overall calorie count.

11. Foods with a lot of sugar added

High added sugar intake is known to be a risk factor for several chronic illnesses, such as type 2 diabetes, obesity, liver disease, and heart disease.

Meals with a lot of added sugar typically have a lot of calories but few other essential elements and are not very satisfying.

Granola bars, low-fat yogurt with additional flavors, and sugary morning cereals are a few examples of meals that may have a significant quantity of added sugar.

When choosing "low-fat" or "fat-free" goods, you should be especially careful since producers frequently add more sugar to compensate for the flavor that is lost when the fat is eliminated.

SUMMARY
 Added sugar has a high-calorie content and may contribute to many chronic health issues. Many goods, even meals with minimal or no fat content, are rich in sugar and should only be taken in moderation.

Chapter 7

what diet results in the highest fat loss.

Should you track your macros or your calories? Reduce calories or carbs? Consume twice as much protein as is advised. Triple? Maybe just connect to a constant protein shake IV?

Finding an eating plan that will burn fat while preserving muscle mass shouldn't be too tough. It's a good thing that the International Society of Sports Nutrition has recently published its position statement, which examines all of the available research to report on how each diet will impact your body composition. Here, we've rounded up the top five diets for achieving a six-pack and explained why they're beneficial for you as well as why they might not be.

THE 5 BEST DIET PLANS FOR WEIGHT LOSS

1. Low-calorie diet
Consuming only 800 to 1,200 calories per day.
Pros: According to the analysis of the study, restricting your daily caloric intake only for the aim of losing weight

quickly while retaining as much lean muscle mass as possible works.

Cons: In our experience, restricting your calorie intake will likely result in considerable internal conflict and tension. Also, we believe that eating should be a pleasure rather than a threat, and 800 calories don't allow many opportunities for taste receptors to be content. Last but not least, reducing your daily calorie intake to this low might wreck your metabolism and hinder weight loss more than switching to one of these other diets could. This is especially true if you are already consuming double to treble this quantity of food. (Curious? These are some reasons why deprivation won't help you lose weight.)

2. Low-fat diet

Receives just 20–30% of one's daily calories from fat; the other 80–70% comes from a combination of protein and carbohydrates, usually with a focus on the latter. Advantages: According to the Institute of Medicine, a low-fat diet (or a high-carb diet, depending on your point of view) is based on the notion that consuming less of the macronutrient that is highest in calories would result in consuming fewer calories overall. Studies have also shown that moving to a low-fat diet can aid in the immediate loss of body fat, albeit not necessarily long-term weight loss.

The old notion that dietary fat is the enemy of body fat is perpetuated by eating in this way. Moreover, it may not be superior to alternative diets: In a research published in the American Journal of Clinical Nutrition, high-protein, normal-protein, high-fat, and low-fat diets were compared. At six months or two years, there was no discernible difference in the groups' rates of fat reduction (though all did result in some fat loss).

Also, although the low-fat group was instructed to maintain a 20% consumption of the macro, actual intake was closer to 26-28%, indicating that for most people, adhering to a rigorous low-fat diet is challenging and may be unachievable.

3. A low-carb diet

Obtaining 15–40% of one's daily calories from carbohydrates, with the rest 85–60% coming from protein and fat.
Pros: Studies demonstrate that switching to a low-carb diet can considerably reduce body fat when compared to a typical diet.

The weight-loss effects are considerably more pronounced when you keep your daily carbohydrate consumption to 20% of your total calorie intake. You can also lower your risk for heart disease and stroke. According to certain studies, low-carb diets are superior to low-fat diets: According to research published in

Annals of Internal Medicine, those who limit their carbohydrate intake lose eight more pounds than those who reduce their fat intake. Your body learns to use fat as fuel when you reduce your carb intake to a certain degree. Although research on the effects of low-carb diets on performance is conflicting, some data shows that those whose bodies adapt to fat-burning relatively rapidly may see an improvement in their endurance performance.

Cons: You have to be patient when you feel lethargic throughout the weeks it takes to become fat-adapted. Training your body to burn fat instead of carbohydrates takes time. Also, not all bodies burn fat as well as others do, so your endurance could never measure up (though, as we said before, others see an improvement here.) If you enjoy sprinting or HIIT, you may need to eat more carbohydrates than other low-fat diets since, without carbs, your body's capacity to produce explosive energy would most certainly drop. Although you'll likely decrease body fat, this type of diet keeps you concentrated on the incorrect macro:
Studies have shown that a low-carb diet's increased protein content, not just its reduced carbohydrate content, aids in weight reduction.

4. The ketogenic diet

Fewer than 10% of daily calories come from carbohydrates, 10%–30% from protein, and 60%–80% from fat.

Pros: The keto diet, while technically a low-carb diet subtype, Is dIstInct because: In addition to forcing your body to become fat-adapted, carbohydrate restriction also causes your levels of ketone bodies to rise, which is essentially an indication that your body is operating on fat. The ketogenic diet induces a special metabolic state called ketosis in which your brain burns ketones rather than glucose, thus improving your mental clarity.

According to the analysis of the study, consuming such a large amount of fat considerably enhances your body's capacity to burn body fat. Also, research demonstrates that keto athletes may reduce fat without sacrificing their strength or power and have a greater VO2 max.
Cons: The same study that highlighted the benefits of being a keto athlete also revealed that individuals on the diet had poorer exercise economies (how efficiently they use oxygen while moving). And although almost every other diet allows for some degree of macro range flexibility, consuming a few extra grams of protein or carbohydrates can cause your body to enter ketosis, so you have to be quite dedicated to reaping the benefits of the keto diet.

Last but not least, you can be struggling because of the minimal protein intake necessary to maintain ketosis: Only 5% more protein on a ketogenic diet quadrupled fat loss, according to a study analysis published in Nutrition, Metabolism, and Cardiovascular Diseases.

5. High-protein diet

What it is: A daily calorie intake of at least 25% protein.
Pros: Of all the diets listed here, increasing your protein consumption has been shown in research after study to drastically decrease body fat and develop lean muscle.
For instance: In just four weeks, men who engaged in sprint interval exercise, strength training, and 2.4g of protein per kg of body weight per day (approximately 1g per lb of bodyweight) in their diet built 1.2kg of lean muscle and lost nearly 5kg of fat.

Research published in the American Journal of Clinical Nutrition supports this. Since protein is so satiating, eating a high-protein diet while reducing calories will help keep hunger at bay and keep your metabolism from falling. Contrary to popular belief, consuming a lot of protein-rich foods won't make you gain weight or damage your internal organs, according to the study analysis.
Cons: Because of the emphasis on protein, it's simple to forget that you need to consume enough fat or carbohydrates to power your activities. So, pay attention to your energy levels and other macronutrients.
The only other drawback identified by the study analysis is that eating a lot of protein might hinder your attempts to gain weight since it is so good at reducing hunger.

Chapter 8

5 Exercises to Achieve Your Body Composition Goals.

Many people mistakenly believe that they have little influence over their physical composition. There is undoubtedly some genetic influence. But, a lot of individuals rely on it and use it as a justification for why they are not physically where they want to be.

What you eat and how you exercise have a huge influence on how your body is made up. This implies that you have control.

Lean mass, which includes your muscles and organs, and fat mass, which is the fat tissue you've deposited throughout your body, make up the majority of your body. You might refer to these things collectively as your body composition.

Just be aware that not all exercise is the same. In other words, jogging and strength training have distinct advantages and have different effects on your body composition. Instead of only doing one type of exercise, they ought to be combined.

Food is not created equally, either.
To control your body composition, it's crucial to control your calorie consumption. Consuming genuine, whole meals, reducing sugar intake, ingesting healthy fats, and obtaining enough protein are all recommended.

What is the perfect composition of my body?

Clarify the goals you have for yourself. What physical goals do you have? Do you want to lose weight and increase muscle? Would you like to gain some healthy weight?

To keep on track, make your goals crystal clear and succinct and remind yourself of them every day. It's normal to be motivated at first, but you need to have a strategy for the days when you're exhausted or feeling down. When you know you're going to require an additional mental boost, prepare ahead of time. To stay in the correct state of mind, watch an uplifting movie, listen to happy music, or even practice meditation.

Many people discover that having an exercise partner helps them stay accountable. Look to them to assist in keeping you on course. Some strategies for maintaining motivation and accountability include joining a gym or enrolling in nearby exercise programs.

Maintain a balanced diet.

You can't out-exercise a bad diet, according to a popular
proverb. It is real. You must consume a portion of
nutritious food to improve your body composition;
exercise alone won't do it.
While there may be a period of adjustment as your taste
buds become accustomed to healthier alternatives, you
will soon be so pleased with how your body feels that
you will start to love giving it the nutrients it needs.

Remind yourself that results take time to manifest and
that you don't have to do everything right away. Wean
yourself off processed junk by incorporating new,
healthier choices gradually. Have fun putting a healthy
spin on familiar meals and trust the process.

How to get your desired body type

Maintain a healthy diet.
Consume a lot of nutrient-rich foods. Try to limit your
intake of sugar and focus on getting adequate protein
and healthy fats.

Be aware of your body.
After consuming anything, do you feel bad? Take note
and make the necessary adjustments. To feel nice, eat.
You won't be misled by your instincts.

Train till you fail.

If you don't push yourself to the maximum, you won't develop and achieve your goals as effectively. You don't know what you're capable of until you reach your physical limit. Although cardiovascular exercise is a fantastic addition to weight training, you will lose fat and weight more quickly if you combine other cardio activities with high-intensity interval training. Remember that your leg muscles are the biggest calorie consumers since they are the largest and most expansive muscles in your body. Your leg muscles need a lot of energy to maintain the force they produce. Hence, performing workouts that activate and recruit all of your leg muscles will maximize the effectiveness of your training. You'll see that the workouts listed below all work your legs or glutes.

The fundamental workouts

You may attain your body composition objectives safely and successfully by including these workouts in your normal program.

1. Burpees

No equipment is necessary. A yoga mat is not required.

Burpees are incredibly effective exercises that work your thighs, shoulders, and core.

How to carry out

Start in the plank position, holding your body up
horizontally with your toes and hands on the floor.
Tuck your knees into your chest, place your feet on each
side of your hands and hold this position.
While standing up, propel your weight via your heels to
jump up. So, one iteration is finished. The objective is to
combine these movements into a rhythmic, continuous
movement.
Finish three sets of ten repetitions.

2. Pushups

No equipment is necessary.
For good reason, this classic exercise motion has been
well-liked in the fitness community for many years.
Pushups bolster your core and improve your shoulders.
How to carry out

Start by lying flat on your stomach in a relaxing position.
When you lift your body off the ground into a plank
posture, use your hands and toes to support your body.
Reverse the process and let your chest touch the floor.
Return your body to a plank posture by pressing your
weight through your palms.
Engage all required muscles by clenching your glutes
together and maintaining a flat back.
Complete five 15-rep sets.

3. Alternating exercises

A treadmill is not required.

Since it keeps your body guessing and raises your heart rate and calorie burning for a significant amount of time, even after you stop exercising, interval training is crucial to achieving your optimum body composition.

How to carry out
Start on a treadmill at 3 mph to get your legs working. Increase the speed to 7 mph after a minute.
After 30 seconds of maintaining that pace, reduce it to 4 mph once more.
30-second portions at 7 mph alternate with 15-second ones moving at 4 mph. Ten to fifteen times should be completed.
Allow yourself extra time to relax between running sets if you need it—no less than 15 seconds. When doing interval training, it's beneficial to wear a heart rate monitor to measure your heart rate. If you are under the age of 55, take care not to go beyond 170 beats per minute.

4. A squat jump with weights

A portable, low weight. A yoga mat is not required.
Your lower body will quickly be sculpted with the aid of this motion. This exercise should feel like it is mostly working your glutes and quads.

How to carry out

Starting in an upright position with your feet slightly wider than shoulder-width apart and your toes pointing forward, support your weight forward in front of you with both hands.
Bring your bottom down to knee height by bending your legs. At the bottom of the action, your legs should make a 90-degree angle. Put pressure on your glutes as you push back up by driving your whole weight into your heels. Keep your shoulders back and your chest out to maintain proper form. Keep your torso from becoming horizontal to the earth. Throughout the exercise, make sure you have a strong hold on your weight. When you perform more reps, you could notice that your shoulders and biceps are growing sorer and sorer.
5 sets of 25 reps should be completed. If you think you can perform more after each set, increase this number. By extending your stance and putting your toes outward, you may do a different variant of the standard squat. Your inner thighs will be the target of this technique.

5. Explosive lunge jump

No equipment is necessary.
If you routinely include this move, your hamstrings, and glutes will be in the greatest form of your life. Your legs will start to feel tight right away, and your heart rate will increase.

How to carry out
Put your feet shoulder-width apart and stand straight up.

Step forward with your right leg, lowering your bottom until your rear leg touches the ground.
Stand back up by bringing your weight down via your front heel.
The identical movement should be done with your left leg.
Despite your temptation to sag, resist it. Keep your abs contracted and your stomach upright.
Make five sets of 30 lunges (15 on each leg, per set).

Chapter 9

How to lose fat and build muscle.
It is frequently asserted that gaining muscle and decreasing fat is incompatible. It might seem completely difficult to accomplish these two objectives since you must eat less to decrease body fat and more to gain muscle.

Nevertheless, it is doable. According to research in the journal Medicine and Science in Sports and Exercise, inactive males were able to improve their VO2 max, a crucial fitness indicator, while simultaneously improving their 1 rep max bench press and leg press.

The Burn Fat and Build Muscle Training Plans
To gain muscle, you'll perform a week of heavy weights with low repetitions, and to burn fat, you'll perform a week of light weights with high repetitions. By training your muscles to be both strong and durable, this technique increases metabolism. When you combine these efforts with our well-thought-out diet plan, you'll expose your body to the necessary factors for achieving your seemingly incompatible aims and achieving the ultimate goal: looking and feeling your absolute best.

The "Gain Muscle" Exercise Program

Do this high-weight, low-repetition workout during weeks 1, 3, 5, 7, and 9. Rest for 60 to 90 seconds in between sets to ensure complete recovery. Constantly aim to lift heavier weights.

Monday
 Abdominal and chest
Weighted bench press
Straight-arm dumbbell press
Angle flies
Dips
hefty sit-ups
crouching cable crunches

Tuesday
Legs Barbell Squats
the dumbbell lunge
Leg press Leg extension Deadlift with a barbell with straight legs
crouching leg curl

Wednesday
Arms Underhand Pull-Ups
Bicep curls and EZ bar curls alternately
triceps extension when lying down

Thursday: Day off

Friday
Abs and Shoulders
Dumbbell shoulder press while seated

Overbent Lateral lifts
the front
rise laterally
cables in a row.
Russian medicine-ball maneuver
dumbbell reversal

Chapter 10

The ultimate fat loss plan.

The game of fitness is highly subjective. You should figure out what works for you if you're serious about losing weight.

With the help of the tools and knowledge provided by FF30X, our premier weight loss program, you can reach your maximum potential. Ask Ralph, please.

Check out the free 24-minute version of the best fat-burning workout to try out the program.

The framework that follows should not be viewed as a strict exercise routine. It may be adjusted to fit any schedule, ensuring that the necessary muscles are used and relaxed at the allotted period.

Day One: cardio
Each repetition should consist of 30 seconds of hard work followed by 30 seconds of easygoing. Repeat five times, then pause for 60 seconds before starting the next aerobic activity.

Sprint five times.
Body weight lunges or five repetitions on the exercise bike

5 jump rope repetitions
5 stair climber repetitions or body-weight squats
Burpees or 5 repetitions on the rowing machine
Jumping jacks 5 times.
That's 30 minutes, but you may cut that time in half by
doing fewer repetitions of each exercise or by only doing
part of them.

Day Two: Upper body strength training
Although you'll need gym equipment for these strength
training routines, you may modify them for use at home.

Try performing each of the following in three sets of
10–12 repetitions. Do as many sets as you can and add
a bit more each day if you can't accomplish three:

Dumbbell rows or lat pulldowns
cable row while seated, or Overbent barbell rows
Triceps extension in the air
Bench press with incline dumbbells
biceps curls
lateral raise cable (can also be done with a dumbbell)

Day three: HIIT
High-Intensity Interval Training is a great technique to
get benefits quickly and requires little time or equipment.

Just concentrate on 20 seconds at your fastest pace,
with 10 seconds in between exercises. Try performing
three repetitions of each of the following exercises,

taking a minute to rest, and then repeating. There
should be 3-5 circuits altogether in this:
Lunges
Push-ups
Jack-knife jumps
croaky legs
Rock climbers
tall knee-ups
Arm jerks
Burpees
Planks

Day four: Lower body strength training
You have concentrated on the upper body. Your lower
body should now be worked on. While many of the
activities in this fat-burning workout regimen use both
the upper and lower body, focusing on the legs can help
you burn more calories and stimulate your metabolism.
Do three sets of 10–12 repetitions of each of the
following exercises:
stepping lunges
Deadlift
Weighted crunches
slurred speech
Backward hack squats
calf lifts while standing

Day five: More cardio
 Finishing your training week with some steady-state
cardio is a terrific option. To achieve this, set aside 30 to

60 minutes, and engage in an activity that keeps your heart rate between 110 and 140 beats per minute.
This can be achieved by running, cycling, swimming, or even quickly walking. Although low-intensity exercise has a smaller calorie burn than HIIT-type cardio, it has been demonstrated to reduce stress levels in addition to having many other positive effects. That's why it's a good idea to incorporate one session a week.

You should be able to carry on a conversation while performing this exercise to make sure you aren't exerting yourself too much and negating the advantages.

The other two days should be reserved for relaxation, although they don't have to fall on the same week.

Chapter 11

Ensuring the success of your body composition strategy!

A lot of folks are afraid to walk on the bathroom scale. It may be incredibly upsetting to exercise and maintain a healthy diet yet still see the same weight on the scale.

But it doesn't imply your efforts aren't paying off just because your body weight isn't changing. Your body composition may be changing, particularly if you are exercising.

Science-based explanations of your body composition and suggestions for improving it are provided on this page.

The scale will tell you your weight, but it cannot reveal the composition of your body.

Everything in your body, broken down into separate compartments, is referred to as your body composition. It is typical to employ two compartments: fat mass and fat-free bulk.

All of your body's fat tissue is referred to as fat mass. Everything else, such as muscle, organs, bone, and fluid, is considered fat-free mass.

You might not notice any changes in body weight if both occur simultaneously.

If you start exercising, for instance, you could put on two pounds of muscle in the first month. You could lose two pounds of fat concurrently as a result of increasing your calorie expenditure through exercise or dietary adjustments.

Your body weight won't change since your fat-free mass rose by the same amount that your fat mass shrank.

If you place all of your attention on the scale's number, you risk feeling defeated or angry because your program "isn't working."

This is only one illustration of how understanding your body composition is considerably more beneficial than understanding your weight.

SUMMARY:
Since you can assess both fat mass and fat-free mass, knowing your body composition is more insightful than focusing only on your weight.
How Would You Evaluate It?

The many ways to determine your body composition are numerous. While some are sophisticated and difficult to use, others are quite basic and straightforward.

Only research and medical facilities utilize the most accurate techniques, which are frequently pricey.

Yet, there are several straightforward techniques you may apply at home to get a sense of whether your body composition is changing for the better.

Measurement of Body Circumference

Monitoring the circumference of various bodily parts is one method.

A flexible tape measure may have been used to measure your waist circumference at the doctor's office.

You can measure the diameter of various body parts like your hips, arms, legs, or chest at home.

A low-cost, flexible tape measure can be used to take these measurements.

A change in circumference might offer you a general notion as to whether your mass is becoming more or less fat or fat-free.

For instance, shrinking waistlines often indicate that you are shedding belly fat.

Fat occupies more area than muscle, gram for gram. This implies that even if your weight stays the same, losing fat may cause your waist circumference to shrink.

Increases in arm circumference may indicate that you are building muscle in your arms if you are lifting weights.

Hence, it is crucial to measure consistently each time to obtain more accurate findings.

Chapter 12

Water and its significance for performance, health, and gas loss.

You are aware of your need for water, and drinking it frequently makes you feel better. So when you drink water, what happens inside your body?

According to the USGS, your body weight is around 60% water, which may surprise you. All of your body's cells, organs, and tissues include water, which is used to support other internal activities and assist control temperature. It's crucial to rehydrate by drinking fluids and consuming meals that contain water since your body loses water through breathing, sweating, and digesting.

Related: 6 Weird Dehydration Symptoms You Should Be Aware Of

The Mayo Clinic states that several variables affect how much water you require, including The recommended consumption is influenced by your geographic region, level of physical activity, and any illnesses or other health issues you may be dealing with.

6 Weird Dehydration Symptoms You Should Be Aware Of

1. Water Guards Joints, Spinal Cord, and Tissues

According to the Mayo Clinic Health System, water keeps the tissues in your body wet and does more than merely quench your thirst and control your body's temperature. You are aware of how it feels when your mouth, nose, or eyes get dry? Keeping your body hydrated enables it to preserve the ideal amounts of moisture in the blood, bones, and brain in addition to these delicate places. Water also functions as a lubricant and cushion for your joints, protecting the spinal cord and protecting it from injury.

2. Water Aids in Waste Removal in Your Body

Your body can eliminate waste through sweat, urine, and feces when you consume enough water. According to the National Kidney Foundation, water aids in kidney function by keeping blood arteries leading to the kidneys open and allowing waste to be filtered out. According to the University of Rochester Medical Center, drinking water is also crucial for preventing constipation. There is, however, no proof that increasing your fluid consumption will treat constipation, according to a study.

3. Water Helps with Digestion

Water is crucial for a healthy digestive system. According to the Mayo Clinic, water aids in the digestion of the food you eat, enabling your body to absorb its nutrients. Water moves into your bloodstream after you drink and is used to digest nutrients. It is absorbed by both your small and large intestines. The National Institute for Diabetes and Digestive and Kidney Diseases states that feces turns from liquid to solid as your large intestine absorbs water. According to MedlinePlus, water is also required to aid in the digestion of soluble fiber. This fiber gels with the aid of water and delays digestion.

4. Drinking water keeps you from dehydrating.

According to the Centers for Disease Control and Prevention, your body loses fluids when you exercise vigorously, perspire heavily in hot weather, get sick with a fever, or have vomiting or diarrhea. It's critical to boost your fluid intake if you're losing fluids for any of these causes to replenish your body's normal level of hydration. To cure various medical disorders including urinary tract stones and bladder infections, your doctor could advise you to drink extra water. Your body will need more fluids than usual if you're pregnant or nursing, so you might want to talk to your doctor about your fluid intake. This is especially true if you're nursing.

5. Water Promotes Optimal Brain Performance

Ever have brain fog? Drink some water. Tiny research on adult Chinese males published in the International Journal of Environmental Research and Public Health in

June 2019 found that dehydration reduces memory, attention, and energy. The scientists note that since water makes up about 75% of the brain, it's not surprising. One explanation for the sensation of confusion? Your body must have a proper electrolyte balance to perform at its best. Muscle weakness, weariness, and disorientation are problems that can result from low electrolytes, according to Gabrielle Lyon, DO, a functional medicine doctor in New York City.

6. Water Maintains the Health of Your Cardiovascular System

A sizable portion of your blood is water. (For instance, according to Britannica, the pale yellow liquid element of your blood called plasma contains roughly 90% water.) According to Susan Blum, MD, founder of the Blum Center for Health in Rye Brook, New York, when you get dehydrated, your blood becomes more concentrated, which can result in an imbalance of the electrolyte minerals it contains (sodium and potassium, for example). For the heart and muscles to work properly, these electrolytes are essential. She adds that since dehydration can drop blood volume and subsequently blood pressure, getting up may make you feel dizzy or lightheaded

Water May Aid in Healthy Eating

It might be simple, but it packs a punch. According to research published in the Journal of Human Nutrition and Dietetics in February 2016, persons who drank just 1% more water per day consumed fewer calories, and less saturated fat, sugar, salt, and cholesterol. A short research with 15 young, healthy volunteers that was published in Clinical Nutrition Research in October 2018 supported the idea that drinking water may make you feel fuller, particularly if you do it before eating a meal.

Do You Need a Lot of Water?

The National Academies of Sciences, Engineering, and Medicine advise that males obtain 3.7 liters (15.5 cups) of fluids per day and women get 2.7 liters (11.5 cups), which can come from water, other beverages, and meals, according to the Mayo Clinic (such as fruits and vegetables). The U.S. Army Public Health Command offers the Urine Color Test for your use in assessing your level of excessive drinking. Examine the color of your urine after using the restroom. You are properly hydrated if it is extremely pale yellow to light yellow. Dehydration is indicated by darker yellow. You should seek medical assistance if your urine is brown or coke-colored.